Recovering from an Injury

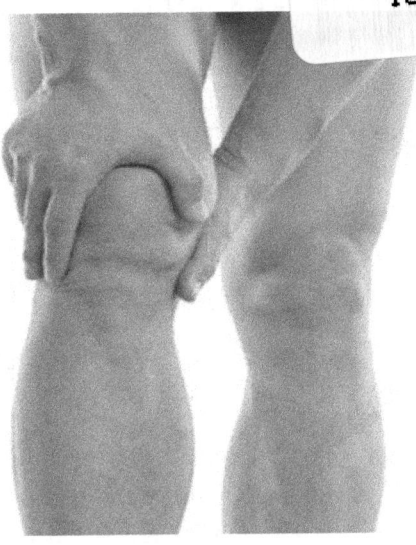

Health Learning Series

M. Usman

Mendon Cottage Books

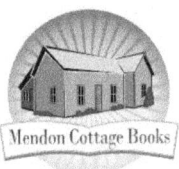

JD-Biz Publishing

Disclaimer

The information is this book is provided for informational purposes only. It is not intended to be used and medical advice or a substitute for proper medical treatment by a qualified health care provider. The information is believed to be accurate as presented based on research by the author.

The contents have not been evaluated by the U.S. Food and Drug Administration or any other Government or Health Organization and the contents in this book are not to be used to treat cure or prevent disease.

The author or publisher is not responsible for the use or safety of any diet, procedure, or treatment mentioned in this book. The author or publisher is not responsible for errors or omissions that may exist.

Warning

The Book is for informational purposes only and before taking on any diet, treatment, or medical procedure, it is recommended to consult with your primary health care provider.

Our books are available at

1. Amazon.com
2. Barnes and Noble
3. Itunes
4. Kobo
5. Smashwords
6. Google Play Books

Table of Contents

Preface

Many have realized the dangers of a sedentary lifestyle. So, we are seeing more people hitting the gym, exercising in the streets, and working out other places. In all fairness, this is a welcome development. Physical activity and good nutrition are the cornerstones of healthy living.

However, we have also witnessed a rise in sports-related injuries. Lack of knowledge on how to exercise properly is to blame for this. If you have been exercising for some time, you probably have had an injury before.

What is awful is that injuries ruin fitness routines. Finding your motivation after you have been sitting for too long is not easy. Additionally, there is the risk of getting out of shape, and some even end up stressed.

Whatever the case, it is important to follow the right techniques for a quick recovery. After all, it is the only chance of getting back into action as soon as possible. A sedentary lifestyle is dangerous and you should not let an injury force you into one.

This book will teach you how you can recover from your injury. The process is not simple or straightforward, as there are a number of things that must be right for a quick and effective recovery.

The first part explains about injuries, their causes, and more. You will then get to the second section, which has information to help in recovery. The last part is about prevention – taking measures keep the injury from happening in the first place is probably the best medicine you can get.

An injury should not make you feel like you are out of ammo. Rather, you should realize that it's time to reload. The majority of injuries can be cured, read this book, and you will know what you should do to get back on track.

Introduction

Chapter # 1: What is an Injury?

A quest to fitness is rewarding both physically and mentally. However, it subjects you to an injury. You can try your best to avoid it, but, sometimes, you are at the wrong place at the wrong time.

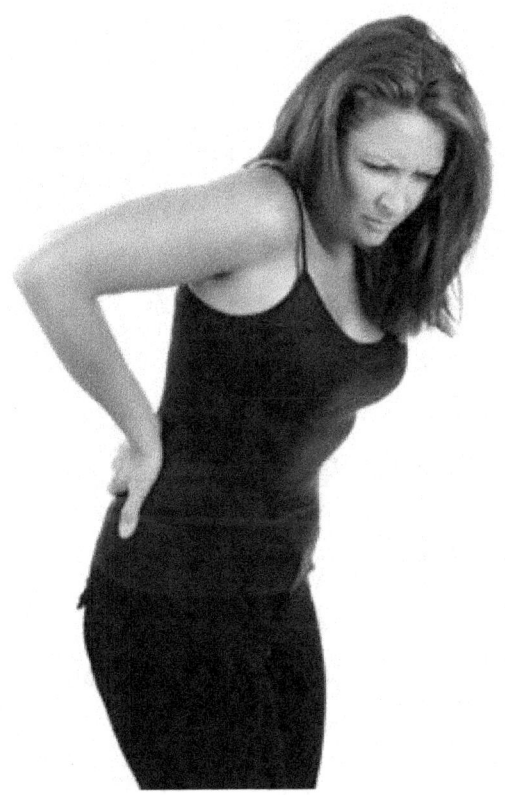

An injury refers to any harm to your bodily organs. This could be the bones, your skin, the neck, hands, back, or any other part. In extreme cases, the results can be fatal, but such incidences are rare. Usually, it's something you can recover from in weeks or months.

Injuries can happen to anyone at any time. Your workouts or how you do them doesn't really matter. Even your level of experience won't make you immune to injuries, although it can reduce the risk to some extent. People have been injured with a simple walk around the block.

When the unthinkable happens, you are forced to sit on the couch until you're fit enough to start exercising again. For others, this can result in depression. Furthermore, there is the fear of putting on weight because of the sedentary lifestyle.

Injuries come in different types, but there are some that are very common:

- Knee injuries

- Dislocations

- Sprains

- Shoulder injuries

- Muscle pulls, strains, and etc.

The severity of an injury depends on the extent of the incident, your experience, help you get, and other factors. Injuries are stressful and it's crucial that you keep a positive mind. Failing to cope with your condition can be more destructive than the injury itself.

Causes of injuries

Here are some of the common causes of injuries:

- ***Inadequate Warm-Up***: By far, this is among the major reasons many end up injured. You wouldn't run a car at full speed without heating the engine first thing in the morning. The same is true with your body. Muscles must be ready with blood flowing to all parts. Failure to do that guarantees you a ticket to the bench.

- ***Using Improper Shoes***: Aerobic exercises, like running, jogging, and walking, require the right shoes. Otherwise, you are susceptible to injuring your foot and legs.

- ***Wearing the Wrong Clothes***: Some exercises demand flexibility from the body, so if your clothes are doing the opposite, you can only expect the worst. But, this doesn't mean you should be exercising naked. Simply buy clothes that give you freedom to move.

- ***Incorrect Technique***: For resistance training, the importance of following proper technique cannot be overemphasized. If you don't know how to do it right, the chances of moving your body in unnatural ways is very high. And so is the risk of injury.

- ***Stress on The Muscles***: Contrary to popular belief, training often does not result in more productivity. Rather, it increases the risk of injury because your body doesn't get enough time to heal.

- ***Pushing Beyond Limits***: We are always striving to reach new heights, as it brings satisfaction and confidence. But, when working out, setting new records must be approached with caution. If it's too heavy for you, try something else. If you can't go another mile, try it some other time.

Chapter # 2: Symptoms and Diagnosis

Not all injuries are as prevalent as falling on your knee or hands. In certain situations, the damage creeps in slowly to the stage where working out becomes impossible. So, you must heed any sign of injury before it advances.

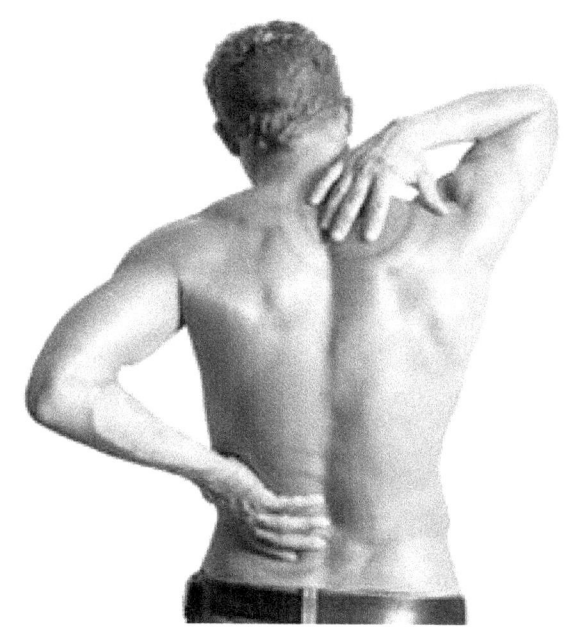

Here are some commons signs:

- ***Pain***: Nearly all injuries are accompanied with pain. You might feel it after the exercise or only when working out. Regardless, this is not a normal part of life. It's an indication that something is wrong, so seek help right away.

- *Swelling*: In addition to pain, you may experience swelling on the affected parts.

- *Tenderness*: With some injuries, you may notice tenderness in some parts of your body.

- *Bleeding*: Losing blood is dangerous so take measures to stop it immediately.

- *Abnormal Shape of Bones and Joints*: Anything unusual in the appearance of your bones or joints should tell you that something is wrong.

- *Bruises*: While not life threatening, it's important to not ignore these. You might have suffered an indirect injury (falling on your elbow might injure the shoulder).

- *Reduced Range of Motion*: If you find it hard to move, you might have an injury that needs to be addressed. You will likely notice this if you are failing to do something you were able to do before.

- *Weakness*: Feeling too weak to finish a workout you have been doing should also tell you that something is out of place.

Diagnosis of Injuries

Seek professional help whenever you believe you have a serious injury. But for bruises or other small damages to your body, you can be your own doctor. When you visit a hospital, medical personnel will use a range of methods to diagnose your condition.

- *Your Description*: This is usually the raw data with any injury. You are asked questions on what happened and your answers are used to determine the type of injury.

- ***Examination***: The affected areas might also be examined for swellings, bleeding, or anything that may be helpful. X-rays are common if a fracture is suspected. But sometimes, this is used to rule out the possibility of a fracture.

If you have been feeling pain for some time, it must not be ignored, no matter how small it may be. Chronic pain can graduate into something serious, so see a doctor as soon as you can.

Recovering From Injury

Chapter # 3: After Injury

Regardless of the type of injury or the cause, you must take necessary measures to ensure a successful recovery. If you keep working out with an injury, you will only make things worse.

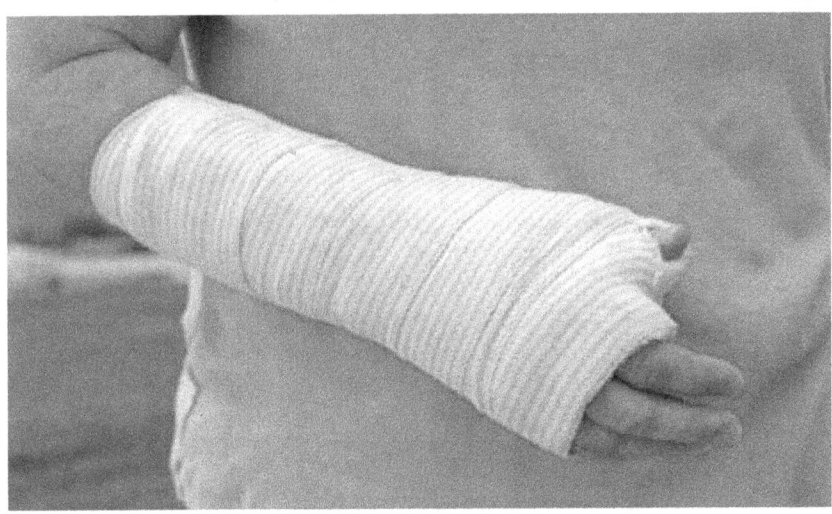

Not every injury deserves to see a doctor. Hurting your finger or wrist can be treated at home, for example. This chapter will give you information to help make the decision of if you need to visit a doctor.

Basically, there are two types of injuries: acute and chronic. Acute injuries are a result of traumatic events like falling, crashing into a friend, and more. They are usually accompanied by sharp pain, bleeding, swelling, etc.

Chronic injuries, on the other hand, are the fruits of abusing your body. So they are also called overuse injuries. Symptoms develop slowly until such a time that working out becomes difficult. Pain, swelling, tenderness, or other symptoms may be felt when working out or when you are finished. Mistakenly, chronic injuries are usually ignored.

Regardless of the type of injury, you must recover fully before returning to action. A reliable method you can use is the PRICE technique.

It stands for Protection, Rest, Ice, Compression, and Elevation. PRICE is mainly effective in the first 48 –72 hours of an injury.

- **Protection**: Once you have identified the affected part, make it a point to protect it from further damage. Otherwise, you risk worsening the situation, which can prolong healing. By far, bandaging works most effectively. Not only does it restrict movement, but it also reminds you of the injury.

- **Rest**: Muscles only recover if given time to rest. So, resist the temptation to get back to exercising, even if your injury is small. You are looking at a couple of days or even weeks off.

- **Ice**: Icing the affected part reduces inflammation and pain. This works by decreasing the amount of blood going to this area. It's most effective when applied within 10 –15 minutes of injury. However, do not try to go for quick gains. If your skin becomes numb, remove the ice and only apply when body temperature returns to normal. Additionally, you should wrap the ice pack in a towel and not put it directly on your skin.

- **Compression**: This also reduces inflammation and pain. A bandage is the best way to achieve this. However, don't make it too tight and if it hurts, loosen it.

- ***Elevation***: Limiting the amount of blood flowing to the affected area lessens pain and swelling. So, raise the injured part above the heart level and gravitational force will do its magic.

After 72 hours, you will start seeing improvement. During this period, you will need more blood going to the injured area. Therefore, you should alternate ice packs with some heat. More blood will bring oxygen and other nutrients to accelerate healing.

In addition, you can take painkillers such as aspirin. If your condition does not improve after a couple of days, see medical personnel, because your injury might be worse than you imagined.

Chapter # 4: Nutrition and Injury

If you have become numb to the phrase "you are what you eat," it's time you changed your attitude. That phrase was true last year and it's still valid today. Food gives us energy, builds our cells, and facilitates a lot of processes in the body. Without it, we would be no different from a rock in the mountain.

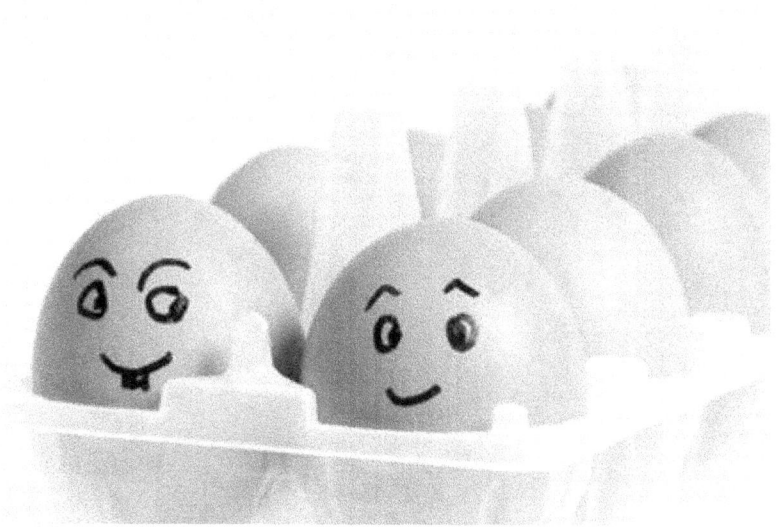

When you have an injury, the importance of food becomes even more prevalent. Having the right nutrients is the only way to speed recovery.

The problem is that many people reduce food intake when injured for fear of gaining weight, since they sit most of the time. But, this is counterproductive. The type of food and not the amount you eat is what makes you gain weight. With an injury, you should increase your intake beyond what is recommended for a sedentary lifestyle. This will give you the necessary nutrients to help in the healing process.

How to Eat

If you have been eating clean prior to the injury, you might already have a huge deposit of nutrients in your body. Mainly, these are vitamins, proteins, fats, carbohydrates, and minerals.

In response to your new condition, you must continue getting all these nutrients.

Fats should be a priority in your diet. However, it should be the healthy ones and not Saturated or Trans fats. Omega 3 fats, found in salmon, walnuts, and other foods, have been known to speed healing.

At the same time, protein must also be beefed up. It is responsible for repairing muscles and building other cells. Without enough of it, your recovery will take an eternity. Good sources of proteins include lean meats, beans, nuts, etc.

You might think that since you are seated most of the times, you will not need a lot of carbohydrates. But this is wrong. Your organs use even more energy than your muscles and if you do not give them enough carbohydrates, they will start using proteins and fats.

As you might have guessed, this will keep you in the bed longer than you anticipated. You can get this important nutrient from vegetables, cereals, fruits, milk, etc.

Adding to all this, be sure to eat a lot of colorful fruits and vegetables. Vitamins are important so make it a point to get lots of them.

However, in this day and age, it is not easy to eat clean – junk is everywhere. No matter your experience, goals, or how you exercise, such food will not get you anywhere. And when injured, your condition will probably take time to improve, because you will not have the necessary nutrients. Even worse, the possibility of gaining weight is always high with junk food.

Cooking at home is the best way to prevent this. Furthermore, you should pay attention to food labels. If you see anything suspicious, go for something healthier.

Chapter # 5: Staying Fit with an Injury

Being injured doesn't signal the end of the road, so don't let it be an excuse for not getting fit. It is very unlikely for anyone to hurt his or her whole body in a workout. That means it's still possible to do some form of exercises.

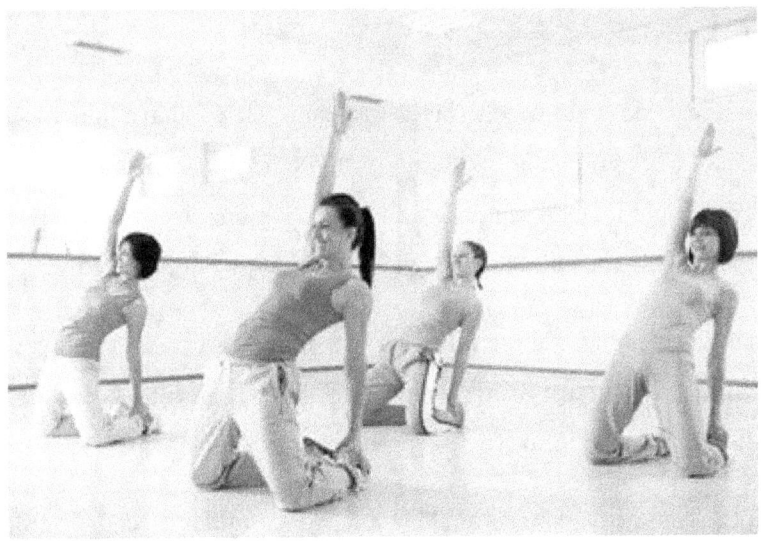

Research has shown that being active helps you recover faster. This is possible, because more blood circulates, transporting nutrients and oxygen to the affected areas. Remember that wounded parts need proteins, fats, and other nutrients for healing.

However, take caution to not increase the injury. If there is a possibility of worsening the condition, give yourself time before you start exercising again.

Besides speeding up your recovery, exercising will ensure that you stay in shape. This is important, as you surely do not want to start from the bottom when you get back to your fitness routine.

Additionally, an injury will give you a chance to try exercises you have never done before. This will help you realize that other workouts are just as fun as the ones you are obsessed with. If you go for resistance training all the time, you will find that running is just as good.

How to Exercise

Your exercise does not need to be extraordinary. If you have injured your hands, any workout that utilizes the legs and other body parts will do just fine. That might include running, walking, or jogging. If it's your legs that are experiencing the pain, think of workouts that do not involve them.

The point is to avoid making full use of the injured area. Although you are allowed to stretch it just a bit, do not get too excited. A little goes a long way. If you find it painful, you are probably doing too much.

If you can't find any exercise suitable for your condition, seek help from a fitness coach.

Chapter # 6: Dealing with Stress

Injured people fall into two categories: those who exercise to keep fit and another group with sports as a career. Those in the former category are not seriously affected. But for those in the latter category, an injury can instantly bring down dreams you built for years. And without necessary intervention, the psychological impact can be devastating.

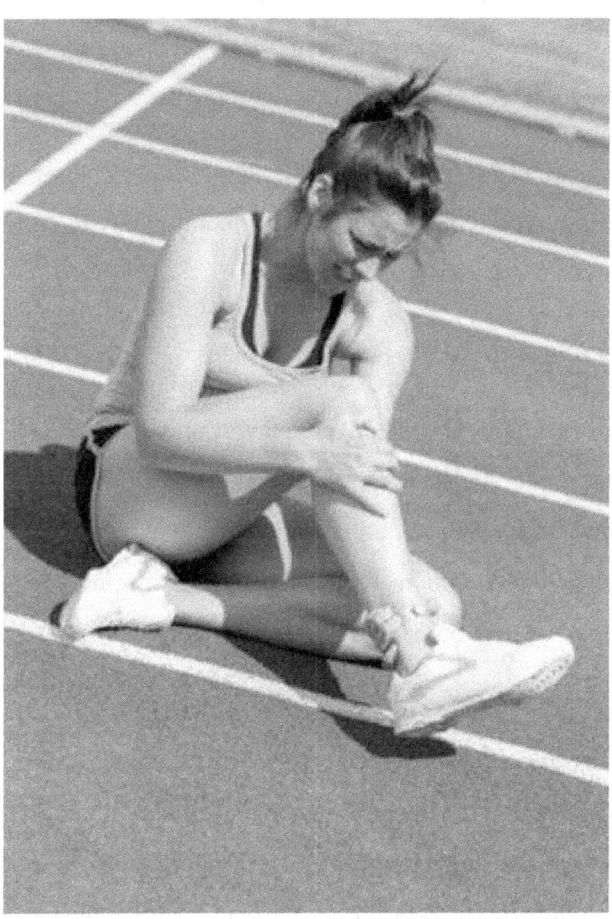

You might have always wanted to be a soccer player, but an injured leg can erase that possibility. If you have a family, you might start thinking of what you will eat, where you will stay, and more. Of all this, fear of a rocky future might set in. As a result, you may become depressed.

Regardless of experience or status, most athletes experience this when injured. Actually, some have even committed suicide.

While not all injuries dictate the end of a career, being on the bench for too long could bring down confidence. So even after recovery, an athlete might not feel the same way. It's not strange to see them trying so hard to prove that they still got it. And this often leads to more injuries.

Other athletes are not so good at doing nothing. So they return to action without making a full recovery. This gives the injury a kingdom to live in and causes even more stress.

Ways of Coping with Stress-Related Injuries

If you keep dwelling on the negative, you will only make the situation worse. Besides, nobody has ever solved a problem by worrying. So look at your condition from a positive angle. With a little patience and discipline, you will realize that the moon and the stars are always there to provide light when the sun is gone. Your situation is no different.

- ***Plan for what you will do if you can't Play Anymore***: Usually, depression comes when you realize that there is no other source of income. Knowing that anyone can be struck with injuries, you must plan now for another career in the event that what you hoped for has been cut short. So if A fails, your plan B will come handy.

- ***Pick Another Sport***: Not every sport requires the same body parts or skills. An injured leg might keep you from soccer or running. But if you think about it, you will find another sport that doesn't demand extensive use of your legs.

- ***Get Support***: Not having a shoulder to cry on is a surefire way to graduate your stress into depression. So talk to your teammates, family, psychologists, and anyone about your fears. After all, a problem shared is a problem half-solved.

Furthermore, it's important to identify stress as it begins. Failure to do that is the difference between you conquering your emotions and vice versa.

Chapter # 7: Making the Return

Getting rid of the bandage or cast doesn't mean it's over. In some instances, the injury might still have some life left in it. This is especially true if you have been your own doctor.

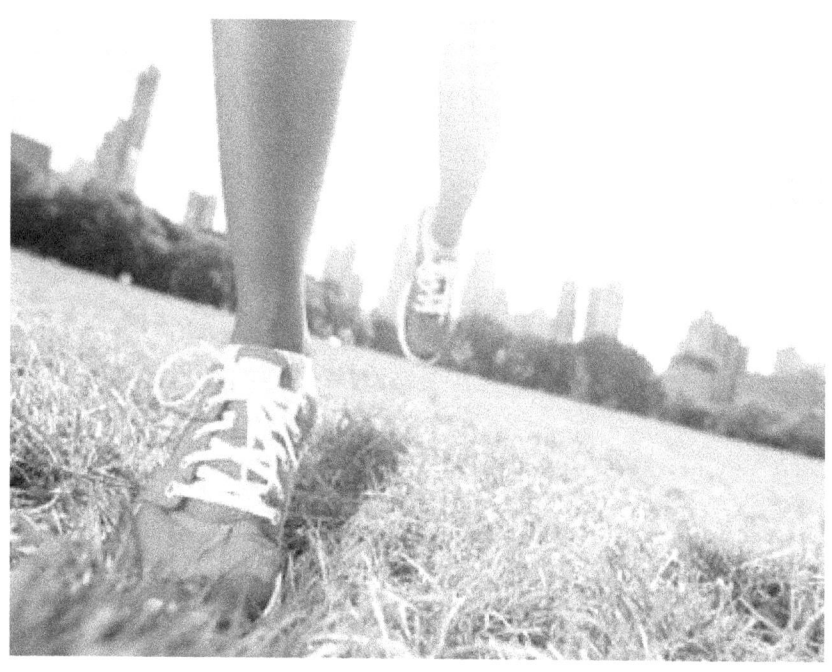

As you already know, it's not a good idea to make full use of your injured part if you have not fully recovered.

Understand the Nature of Your Injury

No one would want to be hit with the same injury multiple times. Unfortunately, in the fitness world, lighting can strike the same place twice. As a matter of fact, some athletes are more famous for their recurring injuries than their work.

To avoid this, you must understand the cause of your problems (killing a snake is best done at the head).

As said in the first chapter, there are a number of causes of injuries. These include using poor technique, not having the right gear, doing too much, etc.

Knowing what is causing your troubles will make it easy to respond effectively. If it's poor technique, working with a coach might help. If you've been doing too much, start giving yourself enough time to rest.

How Long It Takes To Recover

It's impossible to predict the time it will take to recover from your injury. Every athlete is different, and the way your body handles its processes will differ with another athlete. With the same injury, you might be back on your feet in just days, while someone will be laid out for weeks.

Adding to that, recovery time also depends on the extent of the injury. If it was devastating, you are looking at a couple of weeks or months.

You stand a better chance of getting back to action if you have been training during the break. Exercising speeds the healing process and keeps you in shape. However, some injuries might make it impossible to do any kind of physical activity.

The rule is that if you have been out of training for say 2 weeks, it will take you the same amount of time to return to your normal state. However, this does not turn out true every time. I have seen athletes regain their form in less time than they have been out. Interestingly, others find themselves out even after months of training.

Things to Remember When Making the Return

Even with the confirmation that you have recovered, you should approach the first days of exercise with caution. If you go at it recklessly, you will end up with another injury.

1. Take it slowly: It would be foolish to spring into a workout and hit full speed on your first day. You risk sustaining an injury, and you might not feel pain, but that does not mean the injury is gone.

If you are a runner, do not launch into a 5K run right away. For the first few days, just try walking. If that doesn't produce any negative effects, you might then start jogging. If you are still okay with that, you can then start running.

2. Listen to Your Body's Feedback: The first step should make you realize if the injury is still alive. So, pay attention to any clues your body might be giving. If it does not feel right, then it is not right. If you find it painful, something is definitely wrong. Stop immediately and try to establish why you are still having troubles.

Recovering from an injury is meant to bring joy because, again, you will be able to do something you love. But, if you are not careful on your first days or weeks, you will be back on the couch nursing another injury.

Preventing Injuries

Chapter # 8: Warm-ups

Due to ignorance, lack of time, or God knows what, the majority of injuries are a result of not having time to warm-up. The problem is that we sit for too long; we go to the office by car and then sit on a chair staring at the computer all day. Then, we go back home by car and plant ourselves on the couch to watch TV.

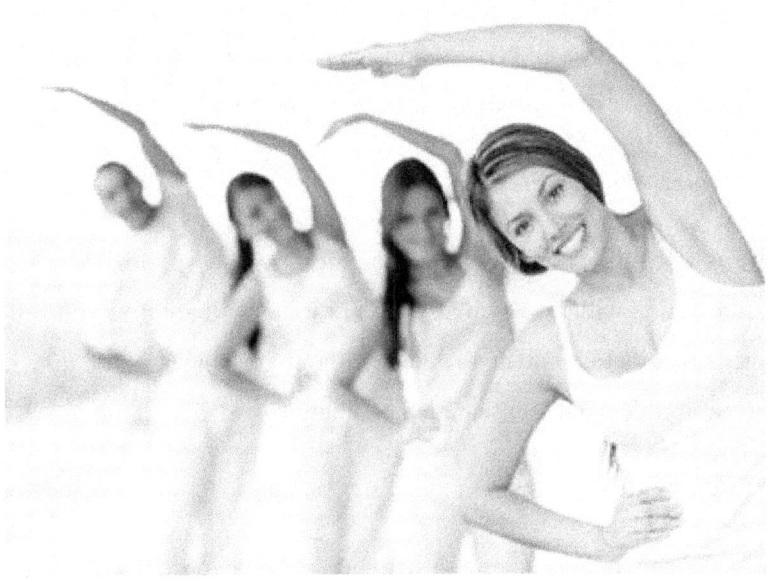

If we lived like in the Paleolithic Era, perhaps there would be no reason for a warm-up. Our ancestors were on the move all the time in search of food and shelter. Being on their feet was a way of life. Fast forward to today and sitting is the way of life.

With this in mind, it's totally absurd to just get up and launch into an exercise. The only thing you will get at the end is an injury.

Here are the benefits of warming up.

1. Loosen Muscles

With muscles stiffened from excessive sitting, the risk of tearing them is very high. But with a warm-up, you can release the tension. After that, you will notice that moving freely is easy.

2. Increases Blood Flow

This is one of the major reasons you must always warm-up. You will increase blood flow to all parts of your body, which in turn will transfer more oxygen. For your information, more oxygen means more energy.

3. Your Joints Will Be Flexible

We are able to move because of the many joints we have. So, if you just jump into action without warming up, your joints will not give you full motion. It will be like moving a wheel without greasing it. Not only will this limit your abilities, but you will also be likely awarded an injury.

How to Warm Up

Warm-ups come in all shapes and sizes. What you choose to go down with depends on your experience, level of fitness, and the type of exercise you plan on doing. The goal is to have a mini version of your main workout. If you are a weightlifter, lifting small weights will do it. Similarly, those going for a run can start off with a jog.

If you have a couple of exercises to do, then make it a point to warm-up every part of your body before the workout.

For example, you can jump rope for 2 to 3 minutes, do arm swings followed by a 3-minute jog, and finish with hip rotations.

A warm-up should last for 5 to 10 minutes.

You might have noticed that some warm-ups can be more challenging than the actual workout. However, this is not a requirement. Your mission is accomplished once your body is ready.

If someone is using your main exercise as a warm up, don't be ashamed about it. We are all different. You are only there to impress yourself so don't go beyond your comfort zone.

Chapter # 9: Using the Right Equipment

Some injuries can be prevented with the right tools. Unfortunately, this is part of the equation mostly ignored. Many focus on technique, nutrition, efficiency, etc. Equipment is nothing more than an afterthought.

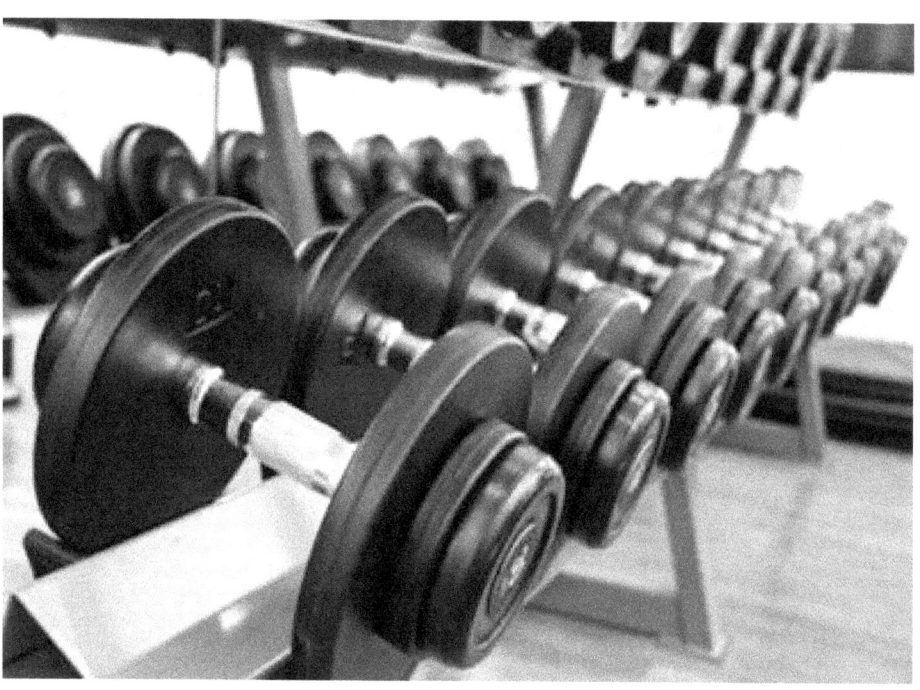

But, if you are serious about preventing injuries, you must first realize the importance of having the right gear. Apart from enhancing your performance, it will also keep you in action.

Each workout demands its own set of tools. So you must first identify the requirements of your exercise. This will help you choose the right equipment.

For example, shoes for weight lift and running will certainly be different. Likewise, what you will need when swimming will not be similar to what you should have when wrestling. Here are some things to keep in mind:

- **Shoes**: With many workouts, shoes are an important part. Your feet take a lot of punishment, so they need the right protection. If not, an injury is likely. While buying any kind of shoes, make sure they're comfortable enough and fit to your feet size. Apart from that, pay attention to the heel – your workouts will determine the type of heel it should be.

- **Clothing**: Your clothes must be flexible. Otherwise, they will restrict movement which can result in injury. At the same time, you do not want them to be baggy, as they will get in the way.

- **Helmets**: If biking or doing sports that risk head injury, head protection is a must. So, choose a helmet that meets safety standards, because injuries to the head can be fatal.

- **Kneepads, ankle braces, etc.**: You must also consider using some form of protection for your elbows, knees, and other joints.

- **Surface**: This is another thing many overlook. Exercising on an uneven platform or one with cracks increases your chances of falling. And this might leave you with a painful ankle, knee, hand, etc. As a precaution, take time to assess the area and identify anything that might cause injury.

- **Weights**: If you are a weight lifter, there is more to consider than just how heavy the weight is. One thing you should keep in the forefront is the condition of the weight itself.

As you can see, the type of workout will determine the equipment you need. Unsure, a quick web search should give you the protective gear needed for your exercises.

Chapter # 10: More Tips on Preventing Injuries

Sometimes, injuries are inevitable. But that doesn't mean you are totally helpless. With a couple of methods, you can keep from them happening. Or at least, reduce their chances.

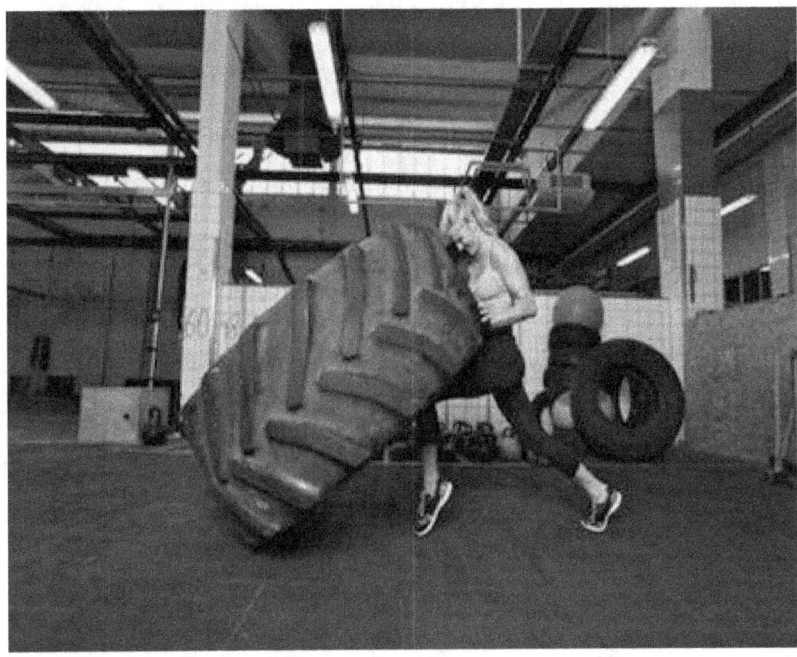

As covered in the previous chapters, it's not only warming up and choosing the right gear that can keep you safe. Your body works in complicated ways and you must keep everything in check to avoid injury. Here some more tips:

- ***Know Your Limits***: It's difficult to resist the temptation of wanting to make quick gains. While the mind is always willing to reach greater heights, often times, the body is not. So be honest with yourself and how far you can go. Digging deeper doesn't always mean you will find the gold. Sometimes, you only dig yourself a hole you won't be able to come out of.

So start slowly and build your momentum with each workout.

- ***Pay Attention to Warning Signs***: If you remember, I said the other types of injuries are chronic. These develop slowly and might take time before you are off the game. To avoid the situation from getting to that point, it's crucial that you take note of the early warning signs. The saying "No pain no gain" is not real, so erase it out of your mind.

If it hurts, your body is trying to tell you that something is wrong. And if you do not address that problem, it will mature into a big injury that will see you sitting on the couch for days or even weeks.

- ***Work with a Trainer***: Using the wrong technique is another leading cause of workout-related injuries. But, if you have a certified trainer, you can learn how to do each exercise properly. Not only that, your trainer will spot mistakes and advise you on how to prevent them. But if you are by yourself, it's easy to develop habits that increase the risk of injury.

- ***Rest***: Others just can't get enough of an exercise and do it more times than what is safe. But this stresses the affected muscles and results in a chronic injury. To avoid this, vary your workouts and give the body enough time to rest. 6 to 8 hours of sleep daily is enough. At the same time, do not exercise every day of the week. Depending on your goals, 5 days or even less should be enough.

Conclusion

Having reached this far, you now know what to do to recover from your injuries. Furthermore, you know the measures you must take to stay safe. It is possible to get back to your previous form, with a little effort.

Soon after your injury, remember to use the PRICE technique. Adding to that, you must watch what you eat and the level of physical activity. These combined will set you on the road to recovery.

If you do not see any change, seek professional help. And when you believe you are fit to start working out again, go slowly. It is easy to worsen an injury if you are not properly healed.

I hope this book has helped to educate you on injuries and how to recover quickly. As always, thank you for reading!

Author Bio

Muhammad Usman is a distinguished medical graduate of Allama Iqbal medical college (AIMC). He is a professional writer who has been in the field for more than 4 years. During this time he has produced 10,000+ articles, blogs, and eBooks on various niches related to diseases, health, fitness, nutrition, and well-being. He is a regular contributor to several journals related to medicine and surgery. He is the editor of several journals and newspapers.

Check out some of the other JD-Biz Publishing books

Gardening Series on Amazon

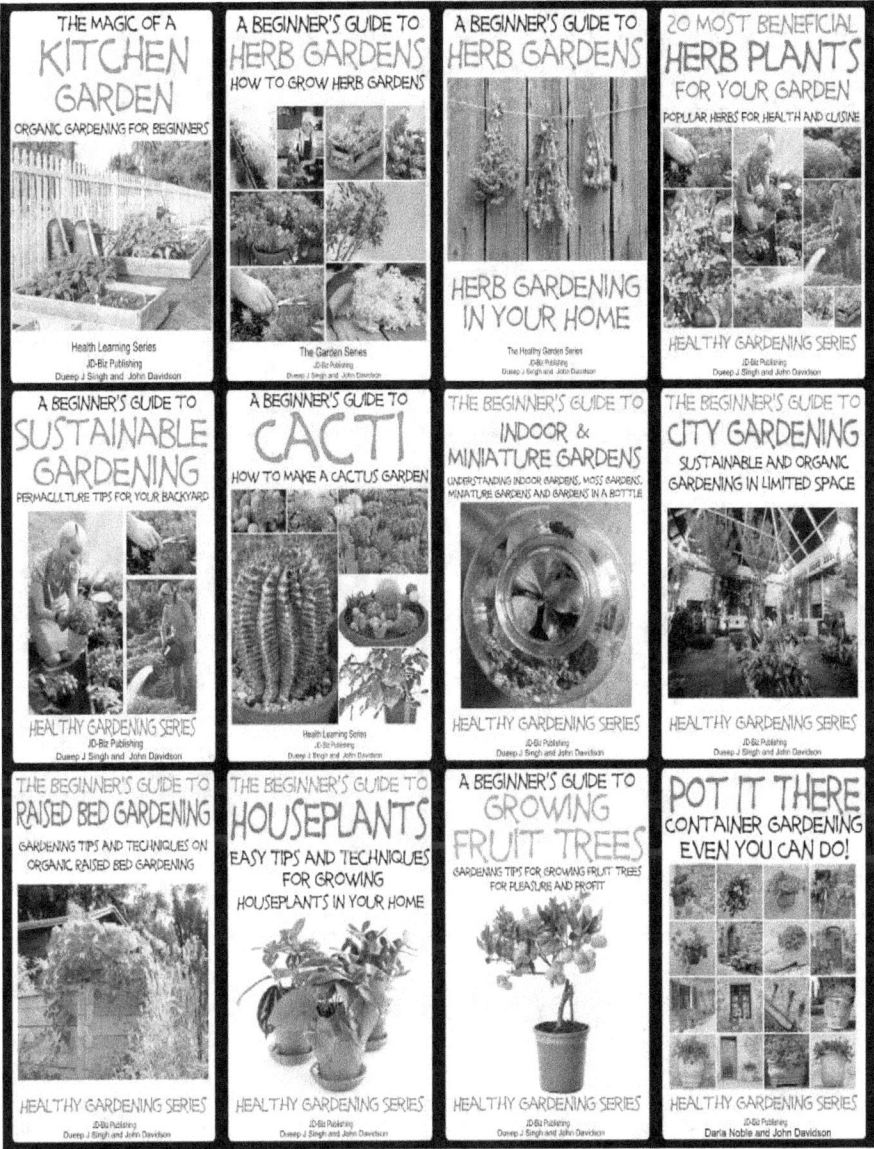

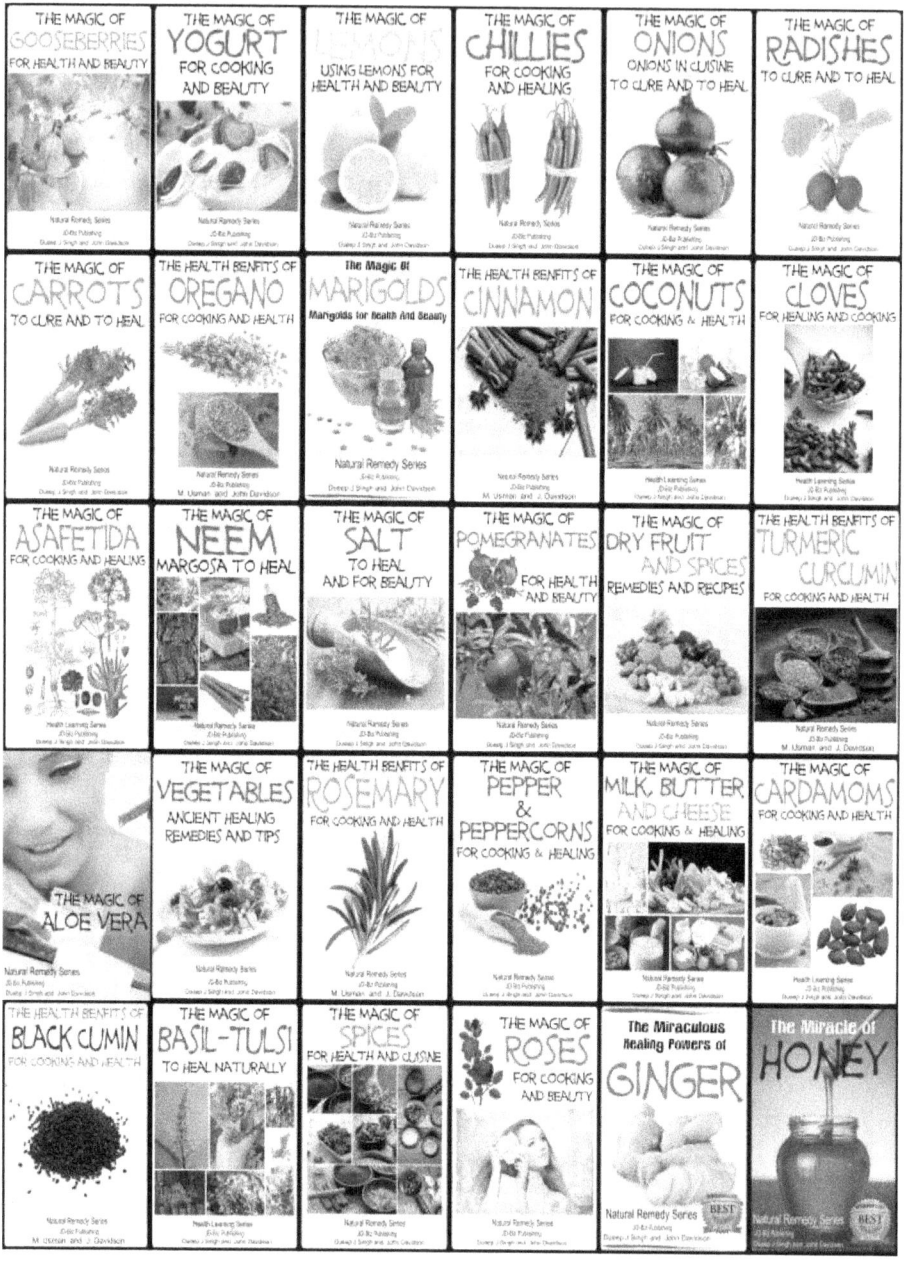

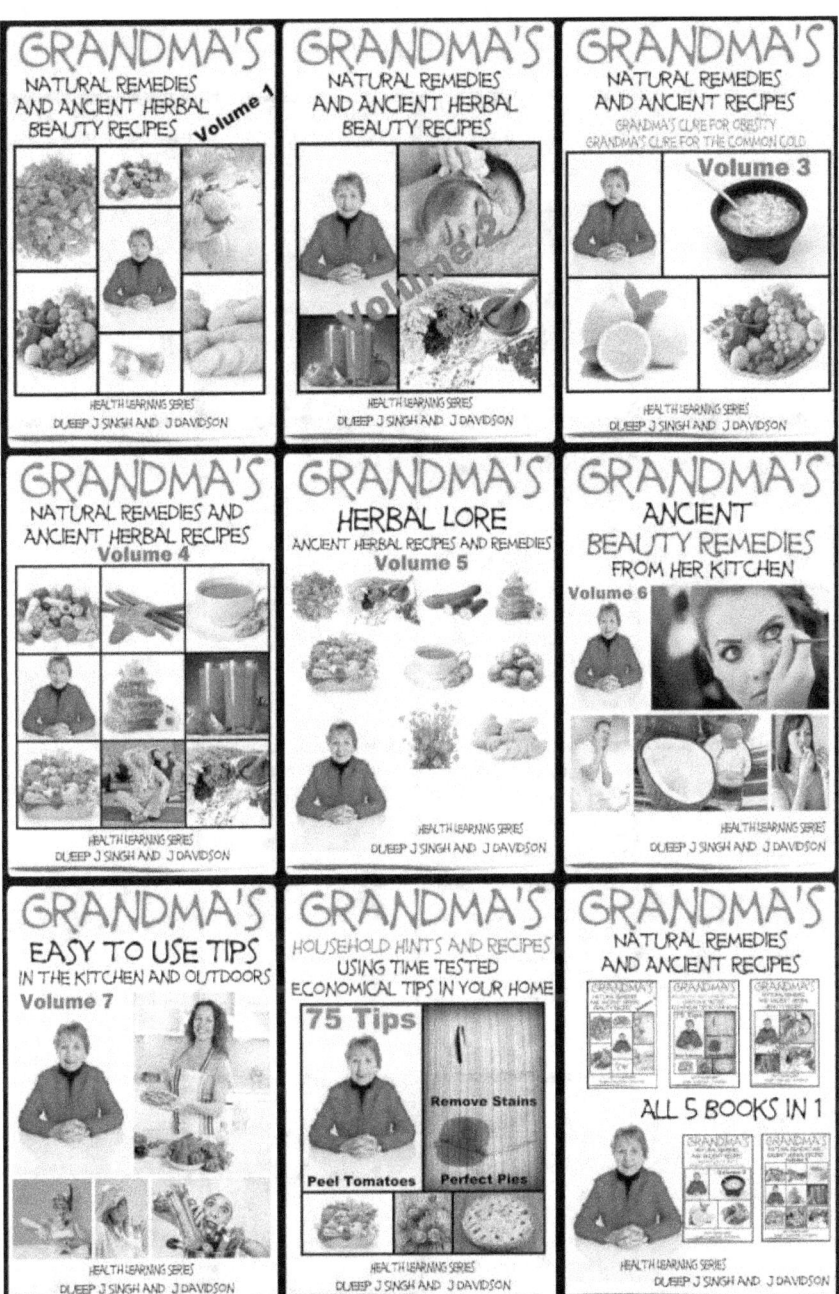

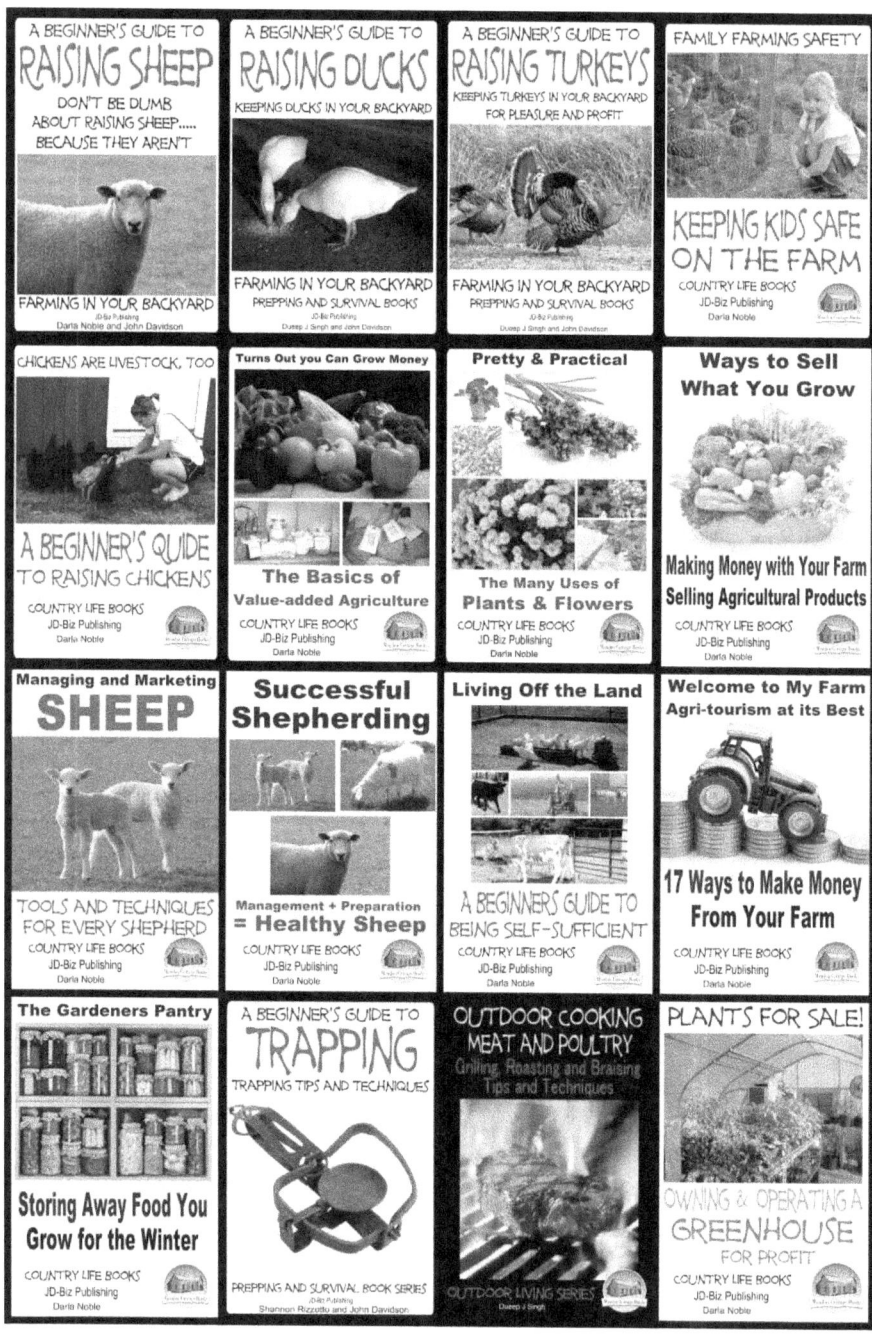

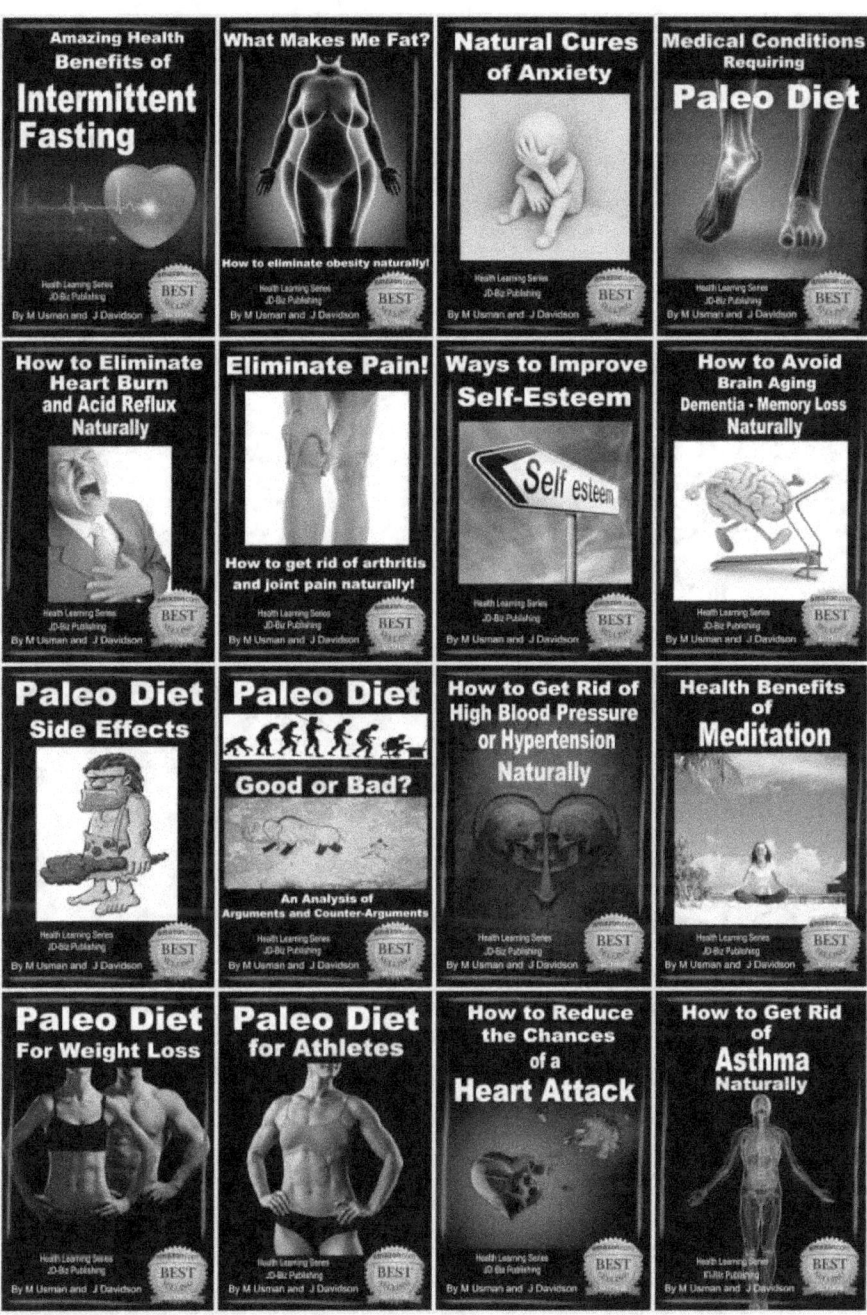

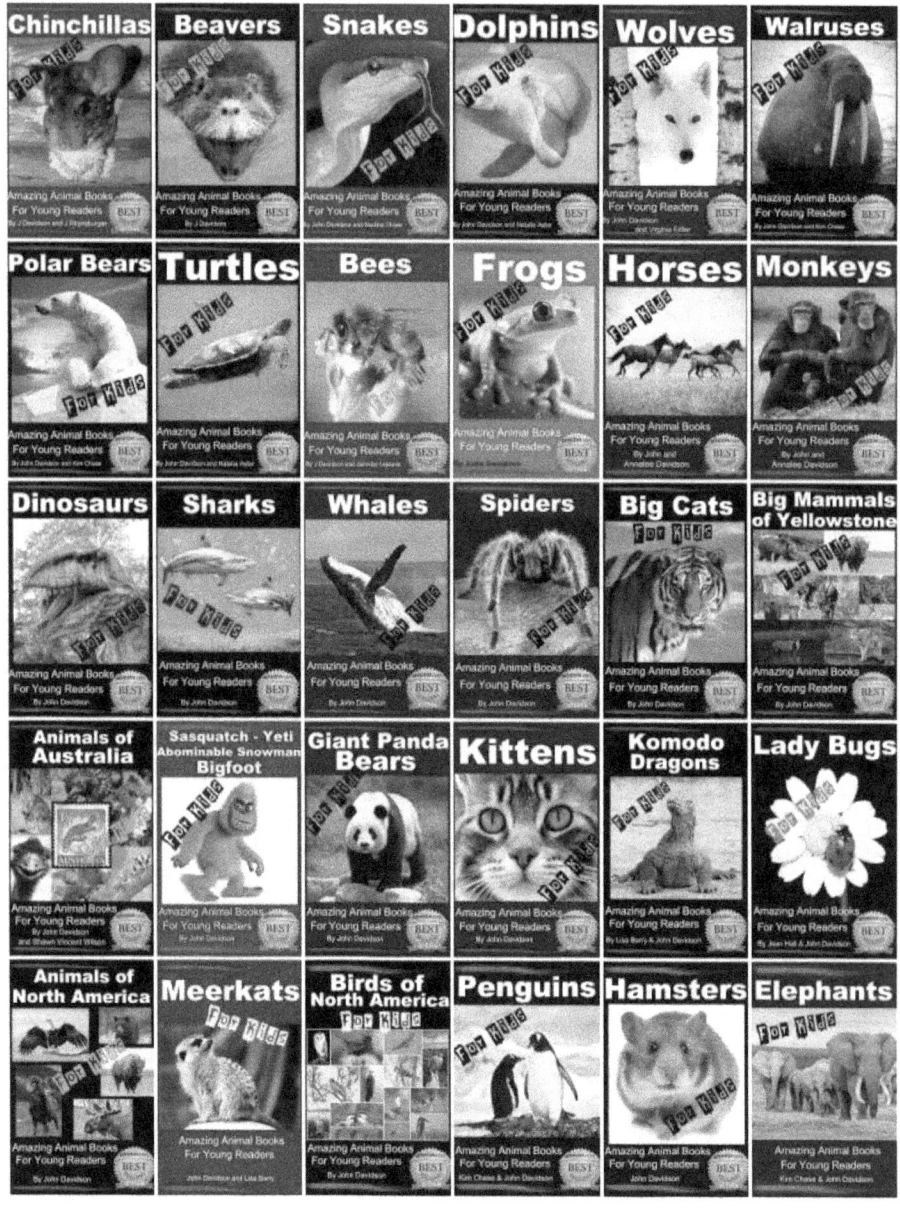

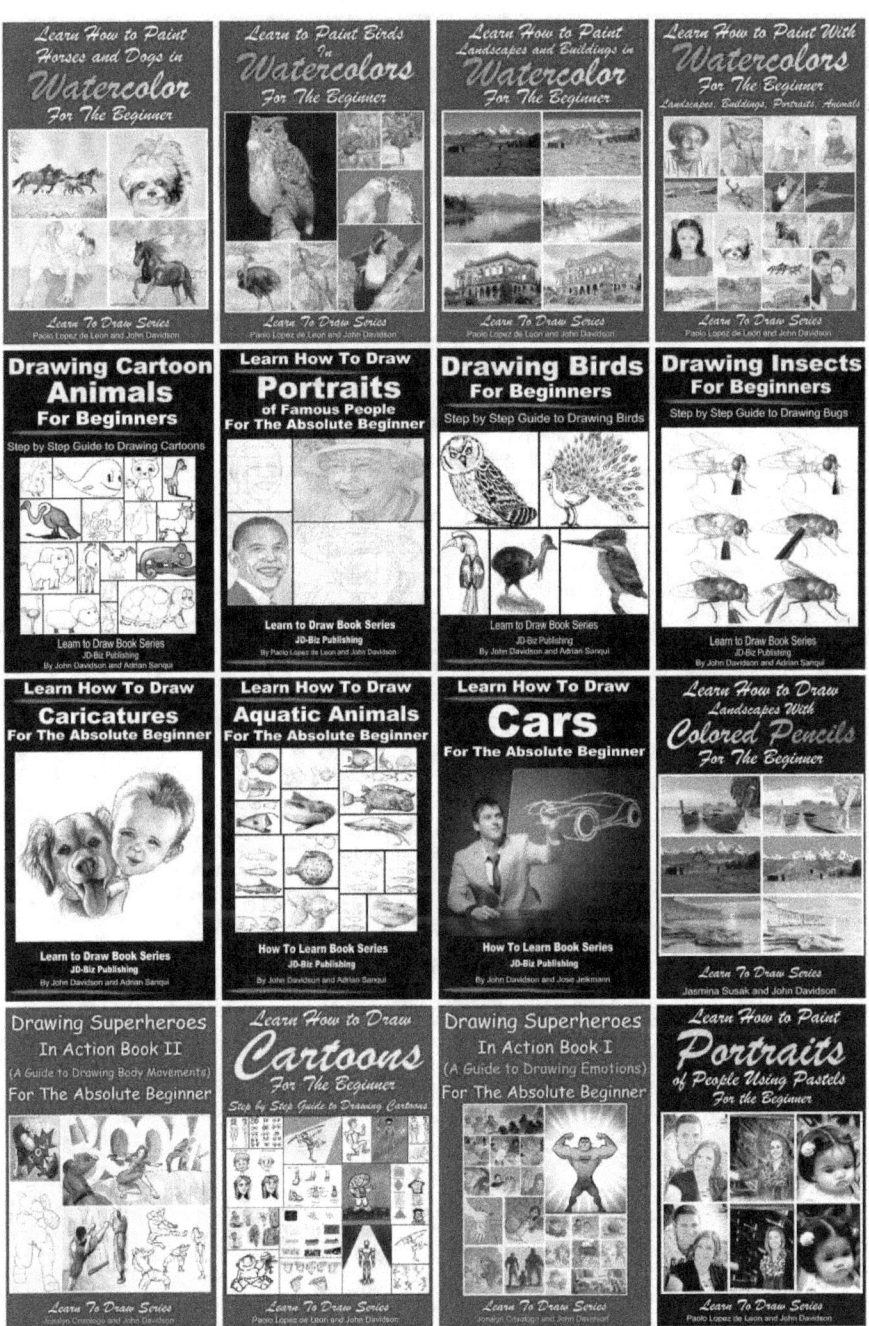

How to Build and Plan Books

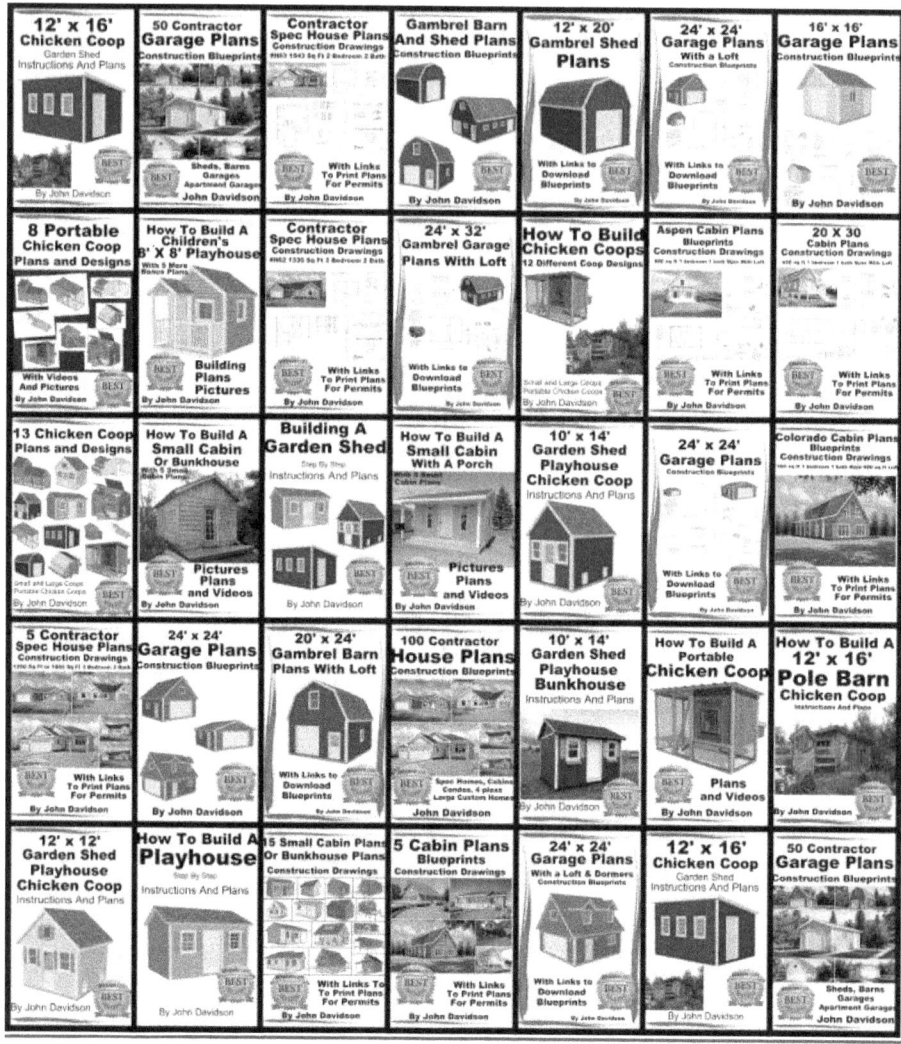

Entrepreneur Book Series

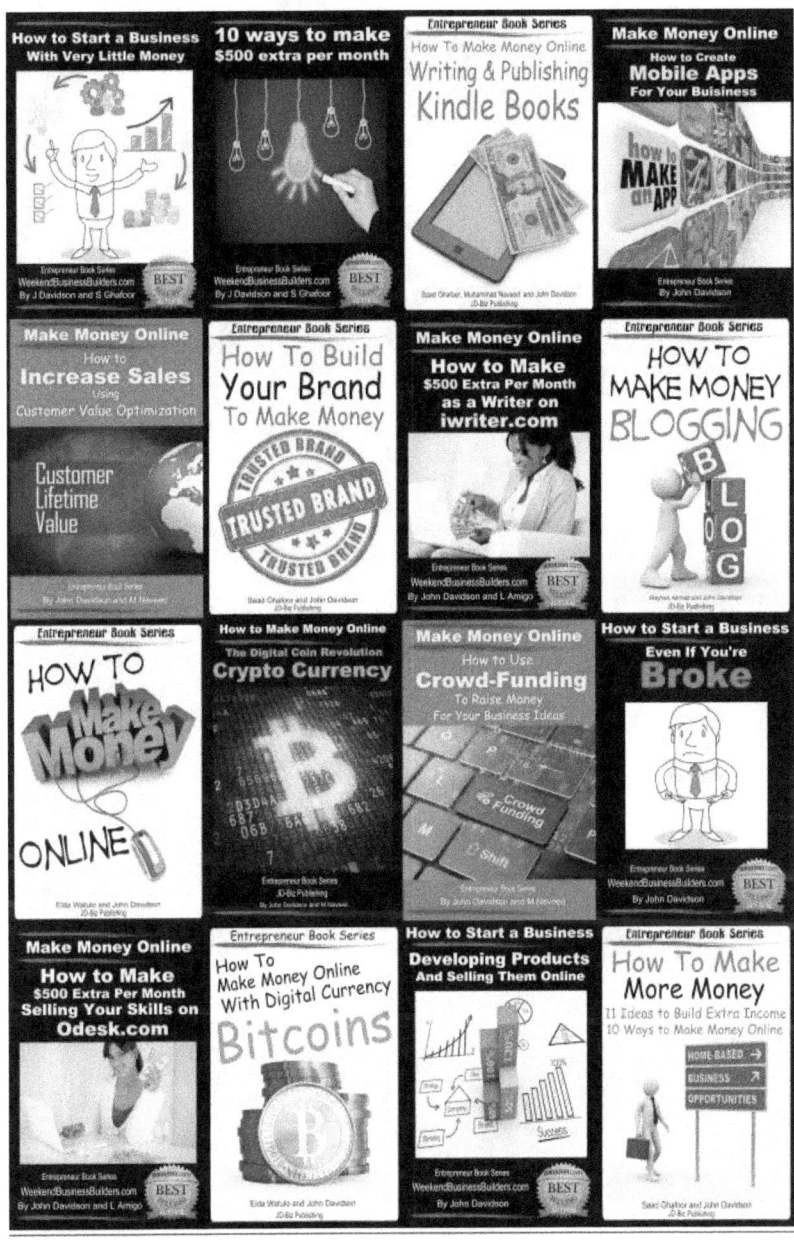

Our books are available at

1. Amazon.com

2. Barnes and Noble

3. Itunes

4. Kobo

5. Smashwords

6. Google Play Books

Publisher

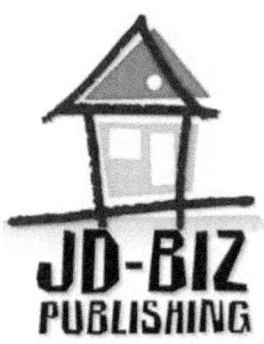

JD-Biz Corp

P O Box 374

Mendon, Utah 84325

http://www.jd-biz.com/

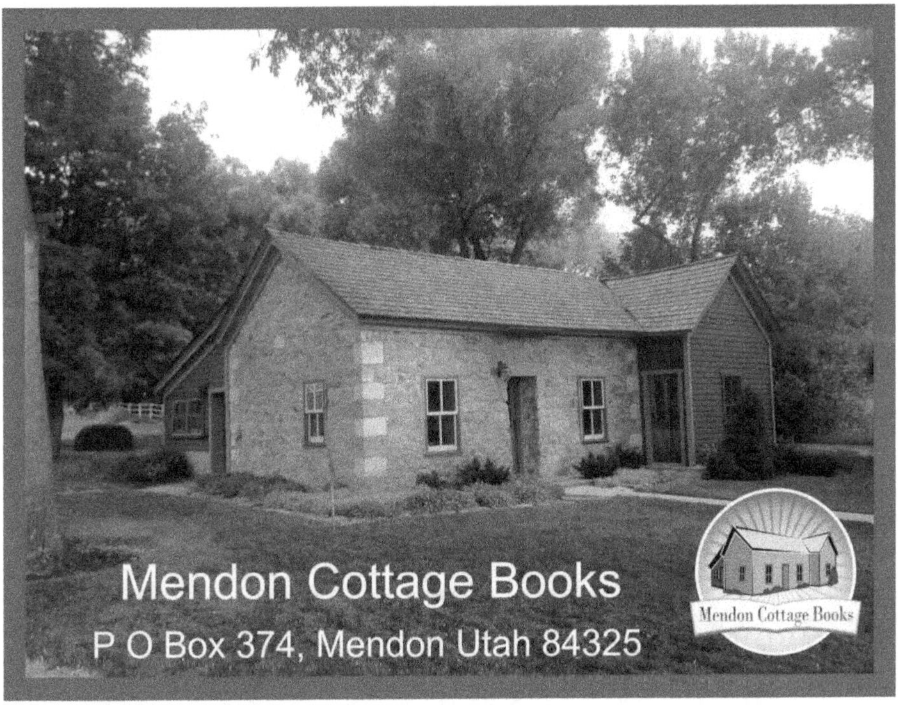

Mendon Cottage Books
P O Box 374, Mendon Utah 84325
Mendon Cottage Books